YEAR 2022

Whitney Samuels

When life gives you lemon make lemonade

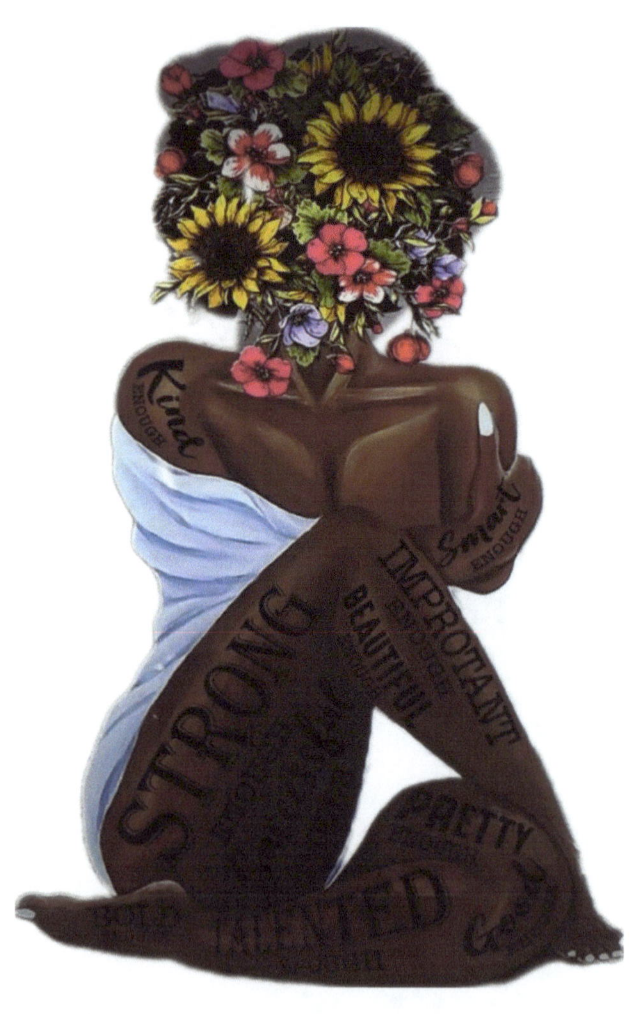

Content

The Start of 2022

Ivy Thompson, a vibrant 22-year-old, started the year with dreams and hopes. Working as an administrative assistant at a thriving marketing firm, she envisioned climbing the corporate ladder. Her mother, Lisa, was her rock, always providing support and guidance. Life was simple but fulfilling. Ivy was Lisa's first daughter which made her want to make her mother proud in everything she does.

Unexpected News

In March, Ivy discovered she was pregnant she did not know how to feel because she had made so many plans and was worried about what her mother would say. She had been in a relationship with her boyfriend, Jason, for a few months, but they weren't planning for a baby. Torn between excitement and fear, Ivy shared the news with Jason and her mother. Jason was supportive but anxious, while Lisa assured Ivy that everything would be okay their reactions and support made Ivy feel better to know that she would not be alone in her new journey.

The Storm Begins

As Ivy's pregnancy progressed, the demands of her job became overwhelming. Morning sickness and fatigue affected her performance, and her boss, unaware of her situation, became increasingly frustrated. By April, Ivy was let go from her job, a crushing blow that left her feeling lost and uncertain about her future. Ivy started to feel depressed she cried most days because she now had to depend on her family which was never in her plans especially with a baby on the way.

A Mother's Farewell

In June, tragedy struck again. Lisa, Ivy's unwavering support system, was diagnosed with a severe illness. Despite fighting bravely, Lisa passed away in July, leaving Ivy heartbroken and alone. The loss of her mother was a devastating blow, compounded by the stress of impending motherhood and financial instability. This news made ivy so stress she ended up in the hospital she could not cope with losing her mother especially when she would need her mother's guidance in her new role as a first time mother.

A Glimmer of Hope

Amidst the darkness, Ivy found solace in her friends and community. They rallied around her, offering emotional and financial support. Jason stepped up, taking on extra work to provide for their growing family. Ivy's resilience began to shine through as she sought out new opportunities, she remembered how hard her mother worked and that was enough motivation as Ivy knew her baby would need nothing but her best,prayers was also her comfort when she felt like she could not go anymore.

Turning the Tide

In September, Ivy discovered a local nonprofit organization that offered support to young mothers. She joined their program, receiving guidance on parenting, job training, and emotional support. This became a turning point for Ivy, reigniting her hope and determination. Ivy discovered her hidden talent of cosmetology though it was tedious standing on her feet which most times lead to them getting swollen fast now with this new discovered talent she rented a shop transformed it into a salon and rented out stations which boosted her earnings while pregnant.

New Beginnings

By November, Ivy had completed the job training program and secured a part-time position at a local bookstore whilerunning her salon. It wasn't the corporate job she once had, but it was a start. She found joy in the simple tasks and the supportive environment. Her confidence grew, and she began to see a brighter future for herself and her little family. Ivy was happy awaiting the arrival of her baby, oftentimes she remembered her mother wishing she was her to see how far she as come and the accomplishments she had gain.

Embracing Motherhood

As the year drew to a close, Ivy gave birth to a healthy baby girl in December. She named her Lisa, in honor of her mother. Holding her daughter for the first time, Ivy felt a profound sense of purpose and love. Despite the hardships, she knew she had the strength to create a beautiful life for her child.The year 2022 had been a tumultuous journey for Ivy, filled with losses, challenges, and unexpected twists. But it also revealed her inner strength and resilience. With the support of her community, the memory of her mother, and the love for her daughter, Ivy embraced a new chapter in her life with hope and determination. The future was uncertain, but Ivy was ready to face it with courage and optimism.

Building a Support Network

As Ivy settled into her role as a mother, she realized the importance of building a strong support network. She joined a local mothers' group, where she met other young moms who shared their experiences and offered advice. These new friendships became invaluable, providing both emotional support and practical help. While working at the bookstore, Ivy rekindled her love for literature and writing. She started a blog to document her journey through motherhood she also was a great business woman her salon became very popular, sharing her struggles and triumphs. Her honest and heartfelt posts resonated with many readers, and soon, her blog gained a following. This not only provided her with a creative outlet but also a potential source of income.

Opportunities Arise

In March 2023, Ivy's blog caught the attention of a local magazine editor who offered her a freelance writing opportunity. This was a dream come true for Ivy, blending her passion for writing with a way to support her daughter. She juggled her business and part-time job at the bookstore with her new writing assignments, feeling a renewed sense of purpose.

Strengthening Relationships

Ivy and Jason faced challenges as new parents, but they grew stronger together. They learned to communicate better, support each other, and share responsibilities. Jason's commitment to his family deepened, and he proposed to Ivy in a heartfelt moment, knowing they had weathered the storm together. They planned a small, intimate wedding for the following summer.ivy could not stop crying wish her mother was here to witness this moment of life, her siblings and her hug and her big brother said that "our mother is watching over us and I know she is proud of everything you had done ".

Paying It Forward

Inspired by the support she received from the nonprofit organization, Ivy decided to give back. She volunteered to mentor other young mothers, sharing her experiences and offering guidance. Her journey from uncertainty to empowerment became a beacon of hope for others in similar situations.

A New Home

With their combined incomes and careful planning, Ivy and Jason saved enough to move into a modest but comfortable apartment. It was a fresh start for their growing family, filled with love and the promise of a brighter future. Decorating the nursery for baby Lisa became a joyous project, symbolizing their new beginning.

Pursuing Education

Determined to create more opportunities for her family, Ivy enrolled in online courses to further her education. She balanced her roles as a mother, business owner, employee, and student, driven by the desire to provide a better life for Lisa. Jason supported her efforts, proud of her dedication and resilience.

A Year Later

By the end of 2023, Ivy's life had transformed significantly. She had a loving fiancé, a beautiful daughter, a fulfilling job, and a clear vision for her future. Reflecting on the past two years, she felt grateful for the challenges that had shaped her into the strong, determined woman she had become.Ivy's story is one of resilience, growth, and transformation. The year 2022 tested her in unimaginable ways, but it also revealed her inner strength and the power of community and love. As she looked toward the future, Ivy knew that whatever challenges lay ahead, she was ready to face them with courage, hope, and an unwavering belief in herself and her family. The journey continues, and Ivy embraces it with open arms, knowing that she has the strength to overcome any obstacle and create a life filled with love, joy, and endless possibilities.

Ivy's blog continued to grow in popularity. Her honest accounts of motherhood and overcoming adversity struck a chord with many readers. With the encouragement of her followers, Ivy decided to compile her blog posts into a book. She spent months refining her writing, adding new content, and seeking feedback from her community.Ivy's book, titled "Ivy's Journey: From Heartache to Hope," was published. The book launch was a significant event, attended by friends, family, and members of the community who had supported her along the way. The positive reception and sales exceeded Ivy's expectations, establishing her as an inspirational author and speaker.

Ivy received several awards for her work, including a community leadership award and recognition from national organizations. Despite the accolades, Ivy remained humble, always emphasizing that her achievements were possible because of the support she received from her family, friends, and community.On a warm summer evening, Ivy hosted a gathering at her home to celebrate her foundation's fifth anniversary. Surrounded by friends, family, and those who had been positively impacted by her work, Ivy felt an overwhelming sense of accomplishment and gratitude. Jason, Lisa, and Liam stood by her side, embodying the love and support that had fueled her journey.

As Ivy tucked her children into bed that night, she reflected on the incredible journey she had been on since that fateful year of 2022. From losing her job and her mother to finding new purpose and building a loving family, Ivy's life had come full circle. The challenges had forged her into a stronger, more compassionate person, ready to face whatever the future held.Standing on the balcony, looking out at the stars, Ivy felt at peace. She knew that her story was not just about her, but about everyone who had supported her and those she had helped along the way. It was a testament to the resilience of the human spirit and the power of community.The end of this chapter marked the beginning of many more. Ivy was ready to continue her journey, knowing that with love, support, and determination, anything was possible. The future was bright, and Ivy was prepared to embrace it, one step at a time.

The End

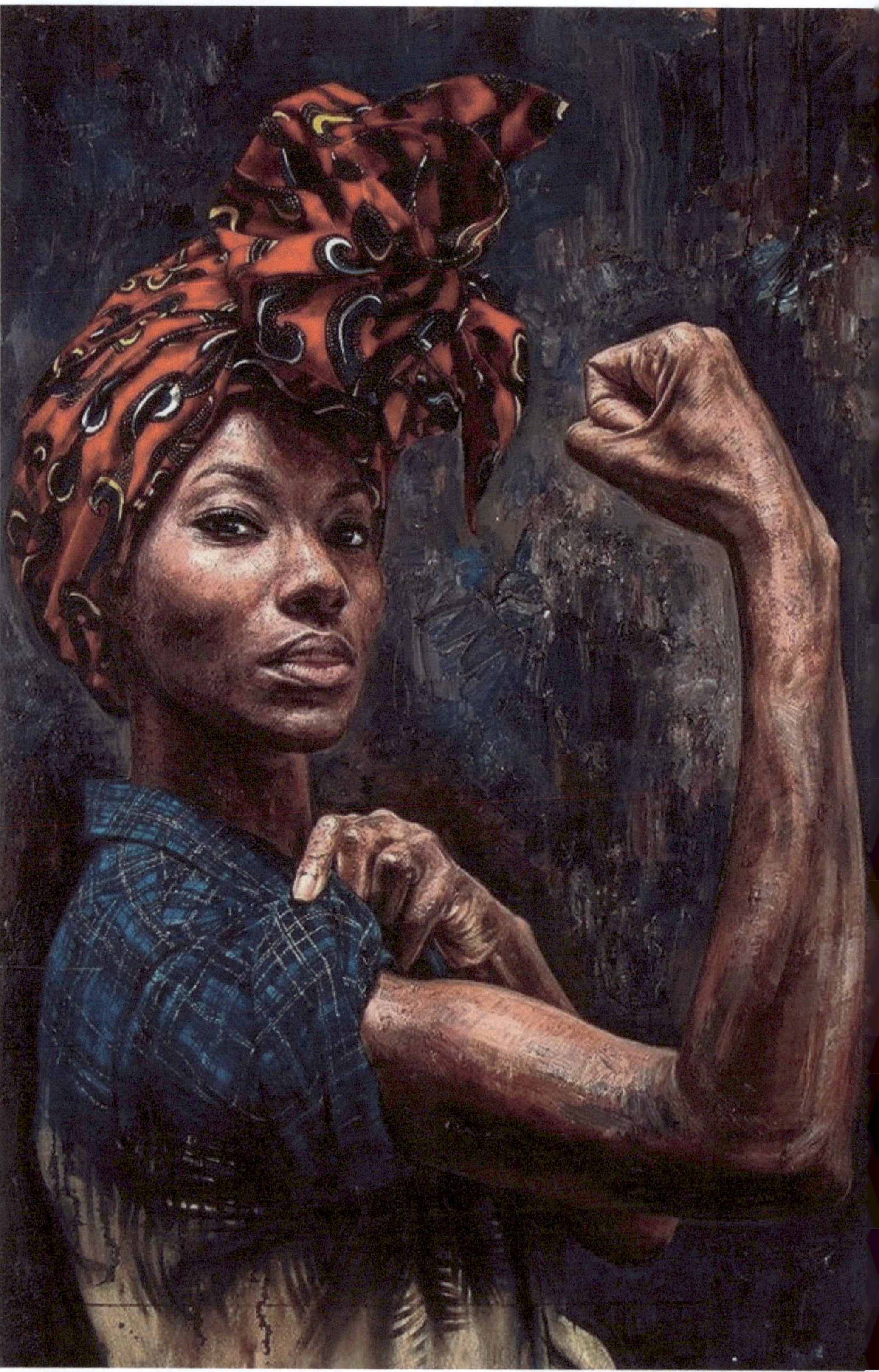

Acknowledgements

This book would not have been possible without the unwavering support of many incredible individuals who stood by me through thick and thin.First and foremost, I would like to thank my mother, Winsome whose strength, love, and guidance continue to inspire me every day. Though she is no longer with us, her spirit lives on in every step I take and every decision I made.

To my children, Elijah and kairo, you are my greatest joys and my driving force. Your smiles and laughter light up my world, and I strive every day to be the best mother I can be for you.I am deeply grateful to my siblings who rallied around me when I needed it the most. Your kindness, generosity, and encouragement have been a beacon of hope. To my readers and followers, thank you for your support and for sharing in my journey. Your comments, messages, and encouragement have been incredibly uplifting, and I am honored to share my story with you.

Finally, to everyone who has faced adversity and emerged stronger, this book is for you. May it serve as a reminder that no matter how dark the days may seem, there is always hope and a path forward. Together, we can overcome anything.With deepest gratitude.

Whitney Samuels

www.ingramcontent.com/pod-product-compliance
Lightning Source LLC
Chambersburg PA
CBHW041805260726
48664CB00034B/425